OXFORD MEDICAL PU

Psychiatric Exam

Mary Robertson March 90

Psychiatric Examination

Notes on eliciting and recording clinical information in psychiatric patients

The Departments of Psychiatry
and Child Psychiatry
The Institute of Psychiatry
and
The Maudsley Hospital
London

Second edition

OXFORD   NEW YORK   TOKYO
OXFORD UNIVERSITY PRESS

Oxford University Press, Walton Street, Oxford OX2 6DP
Oxford New York Toronto
Delhi Bombay Calcutta Madras Karachi
Petaling Jaya Singapore Hong Kong Tokyo
Nairobi Dar es Salaam Cape Town
Melbourne Auckland

and associated companies in
Berlin Ibadan
Oxford is a trade mark of Oxford University Press

First edition published in 1973 under the title Notes on Eliciting and Recording Clinical Information
Reprinted 1975, 1978, 1979, 1982, 1984, 1985
Second edition 1987
Reprinted 1988, 1990

British Library Cataloguing in Publication Data
University of London. Institute of Psychiatry.
Department of Psychiatry
Psychiatric examination: notes on eliciting
and recording clinical information in
psychiatric patients. — 2nd ed.
I. Interviewing in psychiatry
I. Title   II. University of London. Institute
of Psychiatry. Department of Psychiatry
Notes on eliciting and recording clinical
information
616.89'0751   RC480.7
ISBN 0-19-261670-6

Library of Congress Cataloging in Publication Data
Psychiatric examination.
(Oxford medical publications)
Rev. ed. of Notes on eliciting and recording clinical
information/Dept. of Psychiatric Teaching Committee,
Institute of Psychiatry, London. 1973.
Includes index.
1. Interviewing in psychiatry—Handbooks, manuals, etc.
I. University of London. Dept. of Psychiatry.
II. Bethlem Royal Hospital and the Maudsley Hospital.
III. Notes on eliciting and recording clinical information.   IV. Series.   [DNLM: 1. Interview,
Psychological. 2. Medical History Taking.   WM 141 P9737]
RC480.7.P78   1987   616.89'075   87-15213
[ISBN 0-19-261670-6] (pbk.)

Printed in Great Britain by
Express Litho Service (Oxford)

Preface

The first edition of this booklet, originally published in 1973, was written (in the words of the 1973 preface)

to provide guidance for those with little previous experience of psychiatry on the scope and organization of psychiatric case notes and also to ensure that a fairly uniform style and layout are used for the recording of clinical data.

Initially these guidelines were drawn up for the use of registrars at the Bethlem Royal and Maudsley Hospitals, London (familiarly known as the Joint Hospital). Upon publication the 'Orange Book', as it came to be known, quickly found favour throughout the United Kingdom and abroad, and has been reprinted a number of times. In revising the text for this new edition we have discovered how little of the existing material has required alteration. As the booklet has proved particularly useful for trainee psychiatrists starting their careers and preparing for specialist examinations, such as the MRCPsych, this second edition has been expanded with their needs in mind. We have added notes to cover the assessment of elderly and mentally handicapped patients, and patients whose cases have forensic implications. The section on the formulation has been rewritten and enlarged. An entirely new section on interviewing and examining children has considerably increased the size and scope of the booklet, which yet remains a convenient and comprehensive vade-mecum.

We are sure that this expansion is more than justified by the importance now attached to training in child psychiatry and the other sub-specialties both by this Institute and the Royal College of Psychiatrists.

The Institute of Psychiatry,
de Crespigny Park,
London
1987

G. F. M. Russell (Professor and
Chairman) R. J. Jacoby (Editor)
L. B. Campbell A. D. Isaacs
A. E. Farmer J. C. Gunn
M. Prendergast N. L. Holden
E. Taylor

Acknowledgements for the first edition

We wish to give full acknowledgement to those of our colleagues past and present who created this booklet as authors of its first edition: Professor Sir Denis Hill (deceased); Professors R. H. Cawley, R. E. Kendell, W. A. Lishman, M. L. Rutter, and J. K. Wing; Drs J. L. T.Birley, F. Post, and H. H. Wolff.

Acknowledgements for the second edition

We wish to express our sincere gratitude to those of our colleagues who have offered their helpful comments during the preparation of the second edition. In particular we extend thanks to Professor M. L. Rutter and Drs A. D. Cox and S. Wolkind for their major and invaluable contribution to the preparation of Section 10 (Child psychiatry). Special thanks are also due to Professor W. A. Lishman for revising Sections 7 and 8 and the assessment of cognitive function in Section 3 (Mental state examination).

Contents

Introduction

This booklet sets out the guide-lines for compiling the medical notes of psychiatric patients. A high standard of clinical recording is a hallmark of good medical practice and is nowhere more important than in psychiatry. The situation is more complex here than in other fields of medicine because so many different types of information are relevant to the evaluation and management of clinical problems. Many disciplines are involved in psychiatry and there are several contrasting approaches both to theoretical and practical issues. For this reason there can be no final and comprehensive statement about clinical methods which would apply to all patients in all situations, and which would be regarded as appropriate by all experienced clinicians. Differences of emphasis are to be found in different units. The notes which follow should be regarded as a set of general principles which call for flexibility in their application. In practice it will be necessary to be selective and to introduce variations to meet the needs of particular patients and of specialized departments. In the Out-Patient Department, for example, a considerably abbreviated scheme is required for both eliciting and recording clinical information though the principles remain the same.

1

Psychiatric interviewing

The examination of a psychiatric patient resembles a general medical examination in many respects, but there are important differences. These derive partly from the fact that in psychiatry much more attention needs to be paid to psychological and social phenomena, but the main difference arises from the fact that it is the interview itself which serves as the psychiatrist's main tool of investigation.

Psychiatric interviewing is thus a specialized technique of great importance. Three aspects may be distinguished; in different contexts each may assume prime importance, but skilled interviewing aims at incorporating all three whenever possible.

1. The interview is a technique for gathering information. Its objective is to obtain as accurate an account as possible of the patient's illness, the facts of his* background and the significant events in his life, and to gain some understanding of his experiences, and his attitudes towards a variety of people and circumstances. To these ends the examiner must have a clear idea of the range of information he wants, so that he can guide the interview from one subject to another until he is satisfied that everything has been covered. The flow of the interview depends on what the patient says, but the examiner is in control. Nonetheless, even here it is important to be ready to listen to what the patient wants to say, even if this means putting off certain important questions until later. Questions must be framed in a form which the patient readily understands, and presented with tact and sensitivity.

It is particularly important for the interviewer to avoid comments or non-verbal clues which indicate his personal moral feelings. In the face of a history of severely antisocial behaviour or freely expressed hostility, for example, such detachment can be hard to achieve. Nevertheless, the aim should always be for professional objectivity combined with an empathic approach to the patient.

2. The interview also serves as a standard situation in which to assess the patient's emotions and attitudes. If this is to be achieved 'wooden' or stereotyped questioning must be avoided, and the examiner should be warm, empathic, and responsive. He needs to be alert to the implications of the patient's facial expression, his tone of voice, his comments, and his gestures. During the course of the interview, even when discussing relatively straightforward topics, the patient will give many clues about the sort of person he is, and his attitudes and reactions to others (including the interviewer). The examiner should also be able, from his own reactions to the patient, to gain further useful information about him. In fact, the total interaction between doctor and patient is a most important source of information

* The masculine personal pronoun is used throughout for the sake of brevity.

about the patient's personality and mental state, and this interaction should be observed and described by the physician, who, with experience, learns to do so more objectively and skilfully. It sometimes happens, albeit infrequently, that the patient arouses fear in the interviewer. When this occurs the interview should be terminated as it cannot then be conducted safely, objectively, and informatively. If the patient detects fear he may be more likely to react violently. After terminating the interview the position should be discussed with a supervisor or colleague. At some appropriate point the patient should be told what has happened and new arrangements made for the continuation of the interview.

3. The interview, and especially the first interview, fulfils in addition a valuable supportive role and serves to establish an understanding with the patient which will be the basis of the subsequent working relationship. Comments which make the patient realize he is being understood are likely to increase his confidence, while too rigid an insistence on a predetermined form of questioning or ill-timed interruptions will have the reverse effect. In the case of many anxious, suspicious, or hostile patients, the factual detail obtainable at the first interview may need to be limited. Patient, empathic listening is particularly important in such cases and the patient should not be hurried or pressed for answers to questions which he may at first consider irrelevant or embarrassing. Several interviews may be necessary to obtain anything like a complete picture. Anxiety to achieve this too quickly may not only impede the process, but also undermine the relationship on which future interviews and treatment are to be based.

It is important to distinguish between the manner in which information is obtained and the way in which it is subsequently recorded. It is therefore important to retain in one's mind what is ultimately required for a complete history, and at the same time to approach each interview in the light of the patient's present needs.

The *history* comprises data obtained from several sources; it is concerned with the patient's complaints, his recent and remote past, and his present life situation up to the time of admission (or referral in the case of an out-patient). The *examination of the mental state* is concerned with verbal and non-verbal behaviour systematically observed during the interview. Additional observations made elsewhere, either on the ward or in other parts of the hospital, should be recorded under the latter heading, stating their source (informant).

CONFIDENTIALITY

Under ordinary clinical conditions the information collected in the interview will remain scrupulously confidential to the clinical team. However, patients often have fears that information will automatically be given, for example, to spouses or employers. These ideas should be discussed and clear reassurance given whenever possible.

If the purpose of an interview is other than the normal clinical care of the patient, this should be made explicit from the start. Thus, if he is involved in a legal process or under some form of legal duress and information is being collected for a medical report, then it should be made clear to him who else will have access to the report, the nature of the information to be given, and the reasons for divulging it. This is particularly important if the report could be passed to hostile parties.

Firm reassurance about absolute confidentiality should be given only in the most exceptional circumstances and can be guaranteed only by not recording information, which is a dubious clinical practice.

2

History

The history should be compiled from information elicited both from the patient and from one or more informants. Only in exceptional circumstances should the informant be interviewed before the patient is himself seen. The informant's account will not only amplify the patient's reports of factual detail, but also shed light on the patient's relationships within and without the

family. Information from the patient and from different informants should be kept distinct *and recorded on separate sheets.* The
informant's name, relationship to the patient, intimacy, and
length of acquaintance should be noted together with the interviewer's impression of the informant's reliability, and his attitudes to the patient and to the illness. (It may also be important to
record the names, addresses, and telephone numbers of other
potential informants).

The following areas of information should be covered in every
case, although details recorded under each heading may vary
with individual circumstances. The order in which these various
topics are listed is the order in which they usually appear in the
clinical notes. However, when presenting the case to others the
history of the present illness should be read out after the family
and personal history and immediately before the mental state, in
order to put the illness in its proper context. In this case it is often
helpful to give a brief 'thumb-nail sketch' — two or three sentences — before embarking on the detailed presentation.

REASON FOR REFERRAL

Brief statement of why and how the patient came to the hospital.
A note should be made about the referral source and the expecta-
tions of the consultation.

COMPLAINTS

Report by patient, in his own words, not limited to the main
complaints; the duration of each complaint.

PRESENT ILLNESS

A detailed account of the illness from the earliest time at which a
change was noted until admission to hospital. The sequence of
various symptoms should be dated approximately. Note the life
situation and the patient's reaction to it at all relevant times in the
course of the illness. State previous treatment of the present
illness and its effects.

Associated impairments

Describe changes in the patient's relationships with people in marriage, social and sexual life, and at work; alteration in sleep, eating, weight, excretory functions, and drinking and smoking habits; changes in his capacity for making decisions, taking responsibilities, and communicating with others.

FAMILY HISTORY

In cases of fostering, adoption, step-parents, etc., the record should include data concerning the biological and the social family.

Mother

Age, or age and patient's age at the time of her death, and cause of death; occupation; mental and physical illnesses, personality; patient's relationship to her in childhood and subsequently, and reaction to her death; periods of separation in childhood, duration and circumstances.

Father

Data as for Mother; always record details of his occupation.

Sibs

Enumerate in chronological order of birth, with first names, ages, marital state, occupation, significant illnesses, personality (include miscarriages and stillbirths); patient's previous and current relationship with his siblings.

Other relatives

Familial disease, alcoholism, abnormal personalities, mental disorder, epilepsy (say so if information is lacking); note the place and time of psychiatric treatment received by members of the family.

Family atmosphere in childhood

Salient happenings affecting parents and collaterals during patient's early years; emotional relationships within the family;

early stresses arising from emotional or economic causes, including death of, or separation from, close relatives, and patient's age at the time.

PERSONAL HISTORY

Early development

Date and place of birth, birth weight; abnormalities during pregnancy and childbirth including maturity at birth; feeding difficulties; neonatal development, illnesses, and/or fits in this period; developmental milestones, especially general, motor and language development (see also Section 10).

Behaviour during childhood

Persistent sleep difficulties, bedwetting, stammering, tics, or mannerisms; recurrent abdominal pains, fears, periods of misery, shyness, excessive conformity; hyperactivity, serious mischief, frequent fights, truancy, delinquency; play activities and make-believe; ability to make and keep friendships; attitudes to sibs, parents, and strangers, and response to birth of sibs, separation from parents, and to other family crises and bereavements.

School

Age at beginning and end of school life; types of schools, examinations passed or failed; prolonged absences from school and years repeated; specific difficulties, e.g. reading; episodes of bullying or teasing; attitude to peers, teachers, and work; was any special educational need established and if so, at what age? (e.g. prior to starting school or during school years).

Occupations

Age at starting work; jobs held, in chronological order, and reasons for change; satisfaction in work or reasons for dissatisfaction; competence; ambition and prospects; relationship with others at work, detailed inquiry into war experiences and disabilities; promotion in Forces; stability under stress.

Adolescence

Attitude to growing up, to peers, to family, to authority; rebelliousness; drug-taking; periods of depression or withdrawal; fantasy life.

Sexual history

Age at onset of puberty (voice breaking, shaving, menarche) and how regarded; masturbation: age, fantasies, and anxieties; homosexual and heterosexual fantasies, inclinations and experiences, apart from marriage; describe any deviations; current sexual practice — marital and extra-marital; contraception; sexual satisfaction, dissatisfaction and anxieties.

Marital history

Number of previous engagements, associated circumstances; duration of courtship; age at marriage (or marriages); age, occupation, health (past and present), and personality of marital partner; marital relationship, and problems in the past and at present; marriage forced by pregnancy; fidelity of partners; where applicable, date of deaths of spouses, divorces, or separations.

Children

Chronological list of pregnancies (including spontaneous and induced abortions); age and names of children, their physical and mental health in the past and at present time; state place and time of psychiatric treatment received by children; attitudes towards children and further pregnancies; proximity and amount of contact with grown-up children.

Medical history

1. *Illness during childhood*: deliria, chorea, fits, periods of unconsciousness from any cause.
2. *Menstrual history*: regularity, pain, duration, abnormalities; emotional disturbance; date of last period; menopausal symptoms.

3. *General*: illnesses, operations, head injuries, accidents, hospitalizations in chronological order; patient's reaction to these.

Previous mental illness

Details of all psychiatric conditions for which treatment has been received, giving date and duration of illness (specify names of hospitals and doctors). All forms of previous self-injury should be recorded. A special note should be made of all previous suicidal and parasuicidal behaviour, including the precipitating circumstances, the mental state at the time, and the severity of the self injury inflicted. Details of all psychiatric disturbances for which treatment has *not* been received (e.g. behaviour disturbances, alcohol or drug abuse, preoccupation with bodily functions, insomnia, mood variations, pyschophysiological disturbances, anxiety symptoms, etc.). Describe in each case the life situation which prevailed at the time.

Use and abuse of alcohol, tobacco, and drugs

Smoking and drinking habits, including an estimate of the quantities involved recently, and also in the past if significantly different then; attempts to give up and their success; evidence of effects on health, relationships with others, ability to work effectively, and finances; any use of illicit drugs, e.g. cannabis, LSD, amphetamines, cocaine, or heroin; excessive use of aspirin, etc.; dependence on hypnotics or tranquillizers, whether obtained on prescription or not.

Antisocial behaviour

Delinquency or criminal offences, even if never convicted; periods in custody: remand, youth, adult, etc., or on probation; any history of violence or assault; excessive gambling; any history of damage to property, especially firesetting; any conflict with the law about sexual behaviour, drug taking, or drinking. If there is evidence of serious antisocial behaviour, full details about this should be obtained: police and probation reports are very useful. If violence has been used note the circumstances and place (e.g. drunk at home, or an argument in the outpatient department), the nature of any weapon used, the mental state at the time, and the severity of any damage or injuries inflicted.

Life situation at present

Description of the patient's family, housing, social, work, and financial circumstances; satisfactions and dissatisfactions with these; composition of household; difficulties with neighbours; other significant relationships and patient's attitudes towards them; evidence of emotional conflict in family, sexual, or work relationships; recent stresses, bereavements, losses or disappointments, and the patient's reactions to them.

Independent information

To supplement the patient's account is of the greatest importance. This is especially true in potentially embarrassing areas such as the use and abuse of alcohol, and antisocial behaviour.

Mental handicap

If mental handicap is suspected by the interviewer or complained of by the informant, it is important to focus upon those aspects of behaviour, disability, or skills that are causing concern, especially any new disability or increase in pre-existing deficit. Enquiries should be made about the patient's scholastic achievements and social adjustments, e.g. level of reading, arithmetic, and handling of money.

PERSONALITY

The personality of a patient consists of those habitual attitudes and patterns of behaviour, which together with his physical characteristics distinguish him as an individual to others and to himself. Personality sometimes changes after the onset of a mental illness. *If so, a description of his personality before the illness began is required, including information from other informants as well as the patient himself.* The patient's personality is one of the prime determinants of his response to treatment. It is therefore very important to obtain adequate information from a variety of sources. Some of the relevant information will have been recorded under the various headings in the personal history, e.g. how the patient has behaved in different social roles, as a child, parent, sibling, spouse, employee, etc. Other areas of personality functioning are indicated below. Aim to build up a picture of an individual, not a type. Do not merely give a list of adjectives and epithets, which are given here only as guide-lines. *Consider the seven headings listed below and using the data elicited write a description of the patient's personality in non-technical language.*

Attitudes to others in social, family, and sexual relationships.

Ability to trust others, and make and sustain relationships; anxious or secure, leader or follower; participation, responsibility, capacity to make decisions; friendly, warm, demonstrative, reserved, cold, indifferent; secretive, competitive, jealous; dominant, submissive, ambivalent; authoritarian, dependent; aggressive, quarrelsome, sensitive, suspicious, resentful; different attitudes to own and opposite sex; evidence of difficulty in role-taking — gender, sexual, familial, parental, and work.

Attitudes to self

Egocentric, selfish, indulgent; vain, self-dramatizing; critical, deprecatory; overconcerned, self-conscious; attitudes to own performance in different roles; satisfaction or dissatisfaction with self; ambition; attitudes to own health, bodily functions: overconcerned, neglectful; realistic or unrealistic self-appraisal; attitudes to past achievements and failures, to the future, and to dying.

Moral and religious attitudes and standards

Rigid, uncompromising, compliant; easy, permissive, overconscientious, perfectionist; conforming, rebellious; religious beliefs.

Mood

Stable, changeable, swings of mood; optimistic, pessimistic; anxious, irritable, worrying, tense; lively, apathetic; ability to express and control feelings of anger, sadness, pleasure, disappointment, etc., inhibited, open.

Leisure activities and interests

Books, plays, pictures, music, etc., preferred; sport and other leisure activities; creative activities; spends leisure time alone, with one or two friends, or many friends.

Fantasy life

Day dreams, dreams, and nightmares.

Reaction pattern to stress

In suitable cases a life-chart should be drawn up. Ability to tolerate frustration, losses, disappointments, and circumstances arousing anger, anxiety, or depression; evidence for the excessive use of particular defence mechanisms such as denial, rationalization, projection, etc.; evidence of intellectual, educational or emotional deficits in the personality incompatible with roles the patient is called upon to take; evidence for inadequate gratification of biological or social needs through life circumstances or personality inadequacy or deviation.

PREVIOUS RECORDS

Case-notes and/or discharge summaries from other hospitals should be requested as soon as possible — a telephone call to the particular medical records department often expedites the dispatch and receipt of notes. Similarly, other records such as school, probation, and social-work reports should be requested if available. Photocopies of relevant previous records should be placed in the patient's case-file and a brief summary made in the current clinical notes.

3

The psychiatric examination (mental state)

The description of the patient's mental state should record behavioural and psychological data elicited by examination at the time of the interview *as well as observations made in the ward and other parts of the hospital*. It has already been pointed out that there are three aspects to interviewing — obtaining information, observing the patient in a two-person interaction, and giving support. The areas of information that need to be covered in the mental state examination are detailed below. The opportunity should also be taken to record the way the patient reacts to the interviewer and how the interviewer himself feels. For mentally handicapped people whose major disability is a significant but not severe learning difficulty, the normal mental state examination can be applied. In this case, abnormal phenomena carry the same significance as in unimpaired patients and do not simply represent an element of mental handicap.

When describing the mental state of a patient, even very briefly, the term 'normal' is not usually appropriate. Some factual information should be given under as many of the listed headings as possible, so that a clinical judgement can be made of its significance. Such information may also be very useful for future reference.

APPEARANCE AND GENERAL BEHAVIOUR

Give as complete, accurate, and life-like a description as possible of how the patient appears and what can be observed in his behaviour: way of spending the day, eating, sleep, cleanliness in general, self-care, hair, cosmetics, dress; behaviour towards other patients, doctors and nursing staff. Is the patient relaxed or tense and restless; slow, hesitant, or repetitive? Do movements and attitudes have an apparent purpose or meaning? How does he respond to various requirements and situations? Are there

abnormal responses to external events? Can his attention be held
and diverted? Does the patient appear frightened? Does he
appear frightening? (see p. 3).

Does the patient's behaviour suggest that he is disorientated?
Specify orientation if doubtful. Describe gestures, grimaces, and
other motor expressions. Is there much or little activity? Does it
vary during the day, is it spontaneous, or how is it provoked?
Does he, if inactive, resist passive movements, or maintain an
attitude, obey commands, or indicate awareness at all? Do hallucinations seem to modify his behaviour? Even if the patient does
not speak, there should still be a full and careful report of his
posture and behaviour.

TALK

The *form* of the patient's utterances rather than their content is
considered here. Does he say much or little, talk spontaneously
or only in answer, slowly or quickly, hesitantly or promptly, to
the point or wide of it, coherently, anxiously, discursively,
loosely with interruptions, with sudden silences, with frequent
changes of topic, commenting on events and things at hand,
appropriately, using strange words or syntax, rhymes, puns?
How does the form of his talk vary with its subject? Attach or
include in the notes any abnormal written productions. *A verbatim sample of talk should be recorded at this point if there are abnormalities of form.* It should give an adequate demonstration of
formal disorders of thinking such as flight of ideas, thought
block, disorder of logical association, reiterations, perseveration,
incoherence, neologisms, paraphasias, etc.

MOOD

The patient's appearance, motility, posture, and general
behaviour as already described above may give some indication
of his mood. In addition, his answers to questions such as 'How
do you feel in yourself?', 'What is your mood?', 'How about your
spirits?' or some similar inquiry should be recorded. Whenever
depressive mood is suspected specific enquiry should be made
about the following: tearfulness, diurnal variation of mood, suicidal ideas or plans, attitude to the future, self-esteem, guilt,
appetite, weight and libido. Many variations of mood may be

present, not merely happiness or sadness, i.e. such states as anxiety, fear, suspicion, perplexity, and others which it is convenient to include under this heading. Observe the constancy of the mood during the interview, the influences which change it and the appropriateness of the patient's apparent emotional state to what he says. Note evidence of flatness or lability of affect, and specify any indications that the patient is concealing his true feelings.

THOUGHT CONTENT

This should include morbid thoughts and preoccupations. The patient's answers to questions such as 'What do you see as your main worries?' should be summarized. Are there anxieties or preoccupations with the present life situation, with the future, with the past, with the safety of the self or others? Do worries interfere with concentration or sleep? Are there any phobias or obsessional ruminations, compulsions, or rituals?

ABNORMAL BELIEFS AND INTERPRETATIONS OF EVENTS

Specify the content, mode of onset and degree of fixity of any abnormal beliefs.
1. In relation to the environment, e.g. ideas of reference, misinterpretations or delusions; beliefs that he is being persecuted, that he is being treated in a special way, or is the subject of an experiment.
2. In relation to the body, e.g. ideas or delusions of bodily change.
3. In relation to the self, e.g. delusions of passivity, influence, thought reading, or intrusion.

ABNORMAL EXPERIENCES REFERRED TO ENVIRONMENT, BODY, OR SELF

Environment

Hallucinations and illusions — auditory, visual, olfactory, gustatory or tactile; feelings of familiarity or unfamiliarity; derealization; déjà-vu.

Body

Feelings of deadness, pain, or other alterations of bodily sensation, somatic hallucinations.

Self

Depersonalization, awareness of disturbance in mechanism of thinking, or blocking, or retardation, autochthonous ideas, etc.

The source, content, vividness, reality, and other characteristics of these experiences should be recorded, and also the time of occurrence, e.g. at night, when alone, when falling asleep, or awakening.

THE COGNITIVE STATE

This should be briefly assessed in every patient and related to his general intelligence (see the section on Intelligence). In younger patients who are not suspected of cerebral organic disease, the tests mentioned in the following notes for orientation, attention, concentration, and memory should be administered. For older patients see the section on assessment of the elderly patient (p. 34). When cognitive impairment or cerebral disease is suspected, further tests will need to be given from the schema for further examination of patients with suspected organic cerebral disease (p. 23).

Orientation

If there is any reason to doubt the patient's orientation, record the patient's answers to questions about his own name and identity, the place where he is, the time of day, the date.

Attention and concentration

Is his attention easily aroused and sustained? Does he concentrate? Is he easily distracted? To test his concentration and attention, ask him to tell the days or the months in reverse order, or to do simple arithmetical problems requiring 'carrying over' (e.g. 112−25) or subtraction of serial 7s from 100 (give answers and time taken). Give digits to repeat forwards, and then others to repeat backwards (delivered evenly and at one-second intervals) and record how many he can reproduce in each direction.

Memory

In all cases memory should be assessed by comparing the patient's account of his life with that given by others, and by examining his account for intrinsic evidence of gaps or inconsistencies. Special attention should be paid to memory for recent events, such as those of his admission to hospital and happenings in the ward since. Where there is selective impairment of memory for special incidents, periods, or recent or remote happenings, this should be recorded in detail, and the patient's attitude to his forgetfulness and the things forgotten especially investigated. Record any evidence of confabulation or false memories. If the patient confabulates, is this spontaneous or in response to suggestion only? Retrograde and anterograde amnesia must be specified in detail in relation to head injury or epileptic phenomena.

If there is any suspicion of impairment of memory, record verbatim the patient's attempt to repeat a name and address or other similar data, immediately and 5 minutes later.

The following task provides the opportunity for testing free and cued recall separately, and will sometimes demonstrate good learning ability when other techniques have failed. It may also reveal perseveration or confabulation. The patient is told he will be given the name of a flower and asked to repeat it ('the flower is — a daffodil — please repeat daffodil'), then a colour ('the colour is — blue — please repeat blue'), then a town ('the town is — Brighton — please repeat Brighton'), etc. The list continues with items such as cars, days of the week etc., until six to ten items have been given according to the patient's ability. Recall is tested 3–5 minutes later, first without prompting, then if necessary after repeating each category name.

Intelligence

The patient's expected intelligence should be gauged from his history, his general knowledge, and his educational and occupational record. Where this is unknown simple tests for general information and grasp should be given, and an assessment made of his experience and interests. An indirect measure of intelligence might also be obtained from assessing the patient's scholastic achievements by testing his reading, spelling, and arithmetical abilities. A more objective measure can be obtained by using the Mill Hill and Progressive Matrices Tests from which an Intelligence Quotient (IQ) can be derived. If a discrepancy is found between the results of these tests and the level of intelligence anticipated by assessing the patient's literacy and numeracy a learning disorder should be suspected (see p. 67).

PATIENT'S APPRAISAL OF ILLNESS, DIFFICULTIES AND PROSPECTS

What is the patient's attitude to his present state? Does he regard it as an illness, as 'physical', 'mental', or 'nervous', or as needing treatment? What does he attribute it to? Is he aware of mistakes made spontaneously or in response to tests? How does he regard them and other details of his condition? How does he regard previous experiences, mental illnesses, etc.? Can he appreciate possible connections between his illness and stressful life situations, spontaneously or when suggested? Are his attitudes constructive or unconstructive, realistic or unrealistic? Is his judgement good when discussing financial or domestic problems, etc.? What does he propose to do when he has left the hospital? What is his attitude to supervision and care?

THE INTERVIEWER'S REACTION TO THE PATIENT

Here a brief account should be given of the way in which the interviewer is affected by the patient's behaviour. Did the patient arouse sympathy, concern, sadness, anxiety, irritation, frustration, impatience or anger? Did the interviewer find it easy or difficult to control any untoward responses evoked in him or has he failed to do so and, if so, how?

All clinical notes should be signed and dated.

4

The summary

This is an important document which should be drawn up with care. Its purpose is to provide a concise description of all the important aspects of the case, to enable others who are unfamiliar with the patient to grasp the essential features of the problem without needing to search elsewhere for further information.

The first part should be completed within 2 weeks of admission and be drawn up for typing under the following headings:

Reason for referral
Complaint (or complaints)
Present illness
Family history
Personal history
   Childhood
   Occupations
   Marriage and children
   Personality
   Physical illness
   Previous mental illness
Physical examination
Psychiatric examination

The summary of the psychiatric examination should cover all important aspects of the mental state, positive and negative, and be drawn up under whichever of the sub-headings in the main schema are necessary to achieve this. The six sub-headings of personal history listed above should always be included, and others from the main schema introduced as appropriate.

The second part should be completed within 1 week of discharge and be laid out under the following headings:

Investigations
Treatment and progress

Final diagnosis (or diagnoses) and amplifying comment together with the diagnostic code number from the International Classification of Diseases (ICD number)

Prognosis (make a predictive statement related to symptoms and social adaptation, rather than terms like guarded, good, or poor)

Condition on discharge

Further management

The completed summary should be short enough to go on two sides of A4 paper when typed, but only rarely so short that it does not cover one side.

The summary of a readmission should include the full range of categories listed here, unless the last admission was very recent and it has been established that no significant change has occurred in the family history and personal history in the interim.

References to highly confidential matters (criminal acts, sexual revelations, etc.) should be included only if their omission would produce serious distortion of the overall picture. Often it will be preferable to include only a veiled reference followed by 'see notes' in brackets. The summary should identify which professional workers are to be responsible for different aspects of the patient's care in the future.

5

The clinical formulation

The detailed clinical evaluation of an individual patient is known as the clinical formulation and consists of assessment, management, and prognosis. In preparing a formulation the clinician endeavours to integrate all the information that has been gathered on the patient. Thus, the onset and course of the patient's illness is related to the relevant antecedent causal factors. A formulation involves much more than a statement of the basic diagnosis, and should provide a framework within which management can be planned and the prognosis predicted.

After completion of the history, physical and mental state examination the formulation should be written in plain English, not in note form, on a separate sheet. It will vary in complexity from patient to patient, and care should be taken to avoid a mere restatement of the clinical data. The formulation should also be regarded as an appraisal of the patient at one point in time and additional formulations should be written as he progresses or as circumstances change. In general, following admission to hospital two formulations will be written. The first should be completed within 1 week and presented after the history and mental state examination at the first ward round. The second formulation is written when the patient is about to be discharged, and should include the consultant's view of the case, any divergences of opinion, and the patient's response to and compliance with treatment.

It is important to emphasize the need for clear structure and organization in the formulation, and for the account to be narrative in nature and referring constantly to the course of the illness. The assessment concerns an individual patient and general psychiatric knowledge should be introduced only in so far as it is relevant to the particular case. It should not simply be a textbook account of a psychiatric disorder as manifest in an individual.

THE ASSESSMENT

Description of the case

1. Identify the patient: name, age, marital status, occupation.

2. Give relevant background information, selecting data relevant to an interpretation of the genesis of the illness, its form, and content. Give an outline only of: past psychiatric and relevant medical history; family history of psychiatric illness; the patient's personal history and premorbid personality.

3. List the presenting symptoms arranged in chronological order so that the evolution of the illness is clarified.

4. Describe the Mental State Examination, concentrating on salient abnormal findings and stressing normal function when this is important.

5. Physical examination: list abnormal signs.

Differential diagnosis

List in order of probability, with reasons, using the nomenclature of the International Classification of Diseases and its glossary. Restrict the list to those diagnoses which are really possible, and always consider physical disorders.

Aetiology

1. Events: remote, intermediate, recent, maintaining.
2. Type of factor: physical (e.g. genetic, constitutional, physical illness, drugs, alcohol, etc.); psychological (personality structure, psychodynamic); socio-cultural.

MANAGEMENT

For each of the following — investigations, immediate management plans, long-term management plans — consider social, psychological, and biological aspects.

PROGNOSIS

Record both immediate and long-term prognosis.

6

Progress notes

Regular progress notes, *signed and dated*, are a vital part of every case record. They should describe the treatment the patient is receiving (with dates of starting and finishing, and dosages of all drugs), significant changes in mental state, and any important events involving the patient. They should also record the opinions expressed by consultants at ward rounds and case conferences. Although these notes must be detailed enough to convey an accurate picture of the patient's treatment and his response to it, they should not normally contain lengthy ver-

batim accounts of conversations between patient and doctor.
Notes which are excessively long are never read.

A *handover note* should be written whenever the patient is
transferred from the care of one registrar to another, summariz-
ing the salient features and outlining future plans. This is particularly important in the case of out-patients for whom there is
no formal summary or formulation.

7

Further examination of patients with suspected organic cerebral disease

---

Patients with specific or general defects of cerebral function may
or may not be aware of them, and may or may not be able to direct
attention to the disabilities produced by these defects. Examination for such defects should follow a full neurological examination which may indicate detailed inquiry of particular functions.

Testing must not be hurried; *the patient may tire easily and several
sessions may be needed for complete examination.*

The schema of examination and selection of tests must always
be adapted to the needs and difficulties of the individual patient,
and to his intelligence and educational level. The order in which
the tests are offered will often need to be altered when special
disabilities emerge. One disability may have important effects on
performance at other tasks (e.g. receptive dysphasia on tests of
dyspraxia), and due allowance must be made for this in the
administration of tests and the assessment of results.

In all cases, however, it is advisable to adhere to a simple
routine at the start of the examination.

1. First take note of the patient's level of co-operation.
2. Next make a preliminary assessment of the level of
consciousness.
3. Decide whether language functions are intact. Language
functions can be rapidly assessed by: (a) estimating the patient's

verbal ability during conversation and history taking; (b) asking
him to name a series of objects; (c) presenting him with a series of
written commands to point to specific objects; (d) asking him to
write down the names of objects to which you point.

4. Assess the patient's memory, and particularly his ability to
store new information.

5. Use simple screening tests for spatial and constructional
ability, by asking the patient to execute simple drawings and to
copy simple designs selected from those on p. 28.

Assessment of consciousness and of language functions is
essential at the outset, since the interpretation of other tests will
depend upon the patient's ability to co-operate and on the
accuracy of verbal communication between patient and examiner. Memory functions deserve attention next because they
provide a sensitive index of many forms of cerebral disorder.
Screening tests of spatial and constructional ability are necessary
because such non-verbal deficits may otherwise remain
concealed.

The leads derived from the above, together with the patient's
complaints and relatives' observations, will then direct attention
to areas which must be studied in greater detail as described
below. Finally, other functions which have at first sight appeared
to be intact should be examined by simple abbreviated tests.

LEVEL OF CONSCIOUS AWARENESS

Fluctuations in level of consciousness during testing should be
recorded. The relatives or nursing staff should be questioned
about changes from time to time during the day, with specific
inquiry for diurnal variation.

Evidence suggesting a minor degree of impairment of consciousness may have been obtained from the tests of orientation,
attention, concentration, and memory outlined in the general
section of the mental state. The possibility that fluctuation in the
level of consciousness has interfered with registration of ongoing
experience, including that of the interview itself, must be considered. Is the patient alert or dull, wide awake or drowsy? A
simple means of assessing the patient's capacity for sustained
attention ('vigilance') consists in asking him to signal whenever

designated letters appear in a spoken list. Alternatively, he may be asked to cancel all letters of a designated type in a printed script.

If somnolent, can he be roused to full or only partial awareness? If the patient's attention cannot be sustained does he drift back into sleep or does his attention wander on to other topics? Are his eyes open or shut, fixed or following movement? What is the state of his bladder and bowels? The level of consciousness should be documented by defining the nature of the stimulus required to evoke the response and the character of that response.* Evidence for delirium, stupor, or coma should be specified in detail.

LANGUAGE FUNCTION

Motor aspects of speech

Note the quality of spontaneous speech and that in response to questions. Is there any disturbance of articulation (dysarthria)? Is there slowness or hesitancy with production? Does he have difficulty finding words, or use circumlocutions? Does he use wrong words, words that do not exist (neologisms), or words which are nearly, but not exactly correct (paraphasias)? Are there inaccuracies of grammatical construction (paragrammatisms)? Are words omitted and sentences abbreviated (telegram style)? Is speech totally disorganized and incomprehensible (jargon aphasia)? Observe for perseverative errors of speech, echolalia, or palilalia.

Note any discrepancy between what is possible in spontaneous speech and in reply to questions. Minor expressive speech defects may emerge only when the patient is pressed to engage in conversation, to describe his work, his home, or some event in his life. Test whether automatic speech or the naming of serials is better preserved than conversational speech — ask him

---

* The Glasgow Coma Scale assesses three clinical indices, which can be plotted graphically like a temperature chart, as follows.
   1. Eyes open: (i) spontaneously; (ii) to speech; (iii) to pain; (iv) none (no opening).
   2. Best verbal response: (i) orientated; (ii) confused conversation; (iii) inappropriate words; (iv) incomprehensible sounds; (v) none.
   3. Best motor response: (i) obeys commands; (ii) localizes pain; (iii) flexion to pain; (iv) extension to pain; (v) none.

to count to twenty, give the days of the week, or repeat a nursery rhyme. Are emotional utterances and ejaculations preserved when formal speech is defective?

Note. From the phenomenological point of view dysphasic speech may be usefully classified into fluent and non-fluent varieties. Fluent dysphasias in general show normal or excessive output, clear articulation, normal or long phrase length, normal rhythm and inflexion, frequent paraphasic errors, and are produced without effort. Non-fluent dysphasias show sparse output, poor articulation, short phrase length, disturbed rhythm and inflexion, meaningful content when this can be discerned, and speech is produced with obvious difficulty.

COMPREHENSION OF SPEECH

The understanding of speech must be assessed separately, whether or not production is defective. Even if the patient is mute or his utterances totally incomprehensible it is still necessary to determine whether he can comprehend what is said to him. Can he point correctly on command to one of several objects displayed to view? Can he signal his response to simple 'yes — no' questions? Can he carry out simple commands, e.g. pick up an object or show his tongue. Can he respond to more complex instructions, e.g. walk over to the door and come back again, or take his spectacles from his pocket and put them on the table? The understanding of prepositional and syntactical aspects of speech may readily be tested by giving the patient three objects such as a pen, key, and coin, then issuing increasingly complex instructions: e.g. 'put the key on the coin; put the key between the coin and the pen; first touch the key then the coin with the pen', etc.

If comprehension of speech is defective, test whether understanding of written words and instructions is better preserved. Test whether other hearing functions are intact, (e.g. does he exhibit a startled response to noise). Test whether he can recognize non-verbal noises, e.g. clapping hands, snapping fingers, rattling money, or copy the production of such sounds when they are made outside the field of vision (auditory agnosia).

Repetition of speech

Can the patient repeat digits, words, short phrases, or long sentences exactly as you give them? (This involves both motor and sensory parts of the speech apparatus, and also the connexions between the two.)

Word finding

Test specifically for nominal dysphasia by asking the patient to name both common and uncommon objects, and colours presented to him. (This may be the only language disturbance in patients with cerebral damage.)

Writing

Can he write spontaneously and to dictation? Are written productions defective (substitutions, perseveration, spelling errors, letter reversals)? Is copying better preserved than writing to dictation? Is spelling out loud better preserved than spelling on paper? Is the writing of habitual material (signature, address) relatively intact? Are numbers written more accurately than words or letters?

Reading

Test ability to read aloud and to perform simple written and printed instructions. Failing this, can he identify single words or letters? Does he comprehend normally what he reads?

Whenever language disturbances are evident, assess the patient's own awareness of them. *Is he predominantly right- or left-handed?*

VERBAL FLUENCY

Verbal fluency should be separately assessed, even in patients with no other language disturbance, since this is characteristically impaired by frontal lesions. The patient may be asked to name as many words as he can beginning with a certain letter of the alphabet, or as many different girls' names, animals, etc., no matter what letter they begin with.

MEMORY FUNCTIONS

Full examination of memory functions will always be required along the lines set out in the body of the document. Special attention should be directed at recent memory and learning ability. Non-verbal memory should always be tested in addition to verbal memory by asking the patient to reproduce simple figures (see below) after an interval of 5 minutes.

VISUOSPATIAL AND CONSTRUCTIONAL DIFFICULTIES

Test the patient's ability to judge the relationships between objects in space — to estimate distances, to say which of two objects is nearer to him, which is larger, etc. Can he with eyes closed indicate the spatial order of objects in the room around him?

Visuospatial agnosia is often associated with constructional dyspraxia. Test his ability to connect two given dots by a straight line, or to find the middle of a straight line or a circle. Test his ability to draw simple figures (square, circle, triangle). Ask him to copy a series of line drawings of increasing complexity such as those shown in Fig. 1, directly, and from immediate memory. Ask him to draw a house, a clock face and set the hands, to indicate principal towns on a rough map of Great Britain. In such tests and in written productions generally, does he crowd material into a corner of the paper or show unilateral neglect of visual space.

Test ability to construct with sticks or matches a triangle, a square, or to reproduce more complex designs presented to him. Can he assemble a simple jigsaw puzzle or re-assemble a piece of

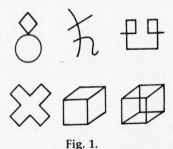

Fig. 1.

paper cut into fragments? If available, test his ability to reproduce patterns with Koh's blocks.

VISUAL AGNOSIA

Can the patient describe what he sees, and identify objects and persons? Ask him to name a particular object in a group exposed to view, to describe its use, or if dysphasic to indicate its use. (If he fails, test whether he can identify it by touch.) Ask him to name the colours of objects. Ask him to describe a meaningful situation in a picture shown to him. Is his recognition of faces defective (prosopagnosia)? Ask him to point out a named person known to him among a group, or to name photographs or relatives or well-known public figures.

DYSPRAXIA

Test the patient's ability to carry out purposeful movements to command, e.g. holding out arms, crossing legs, showing teeth, screwing up eyes, nodding head. Test each hand separately for opening and closing the hand, opposition of thumb and little finger, pronation and supination. Test the patient's ability to carry out complex co-ordinated sequences of movements to command, e.g. light a match, wind a watch, fold paper and put it in an envelope. (Several varieties of dyspraxia are sometimes recognized — limb kinetic, ideomotor, and ideational.)

OTHER DISTURBANCES OF CORTICAL FUNCTION

Number functions

Can the patient read or write numbers of two or more digits? Can he count objects and guess without counting the number of matches laid before him? Assess ability to handle number concepts — addition, subtraction, multiplication, division — in relation to his education and occupational background. Assess ability to handle money correctly.

Topographical disorientation

Does the patient find his way easily about the ward when he would be expected to do so? Does he confuse his bed with other people's? Can he describe the relationships between parts of the ward or of his own house, can he describe the route from home to hospital? If necessary test his ability to follow, on command, a simple route in the ward or hospital.

Right–left disorientation

Can he point on command to objects around him on the right and on the left? Ask him to move, on command, right and left parts of the body, to point to individual parts on the right and on the left side of his own body, and of the examiner sitting opposite him. Can he perform complex instructions like 'touch your right ear with your left hand', 'pick up the left hand match with your left hand and place it in my right hand'?

Body image disturbances

These may include any of the following.

Finger agnosia
Ask the patient to name, move on command or point to individual fingers - his own and the examiner's.

Disturbances of identification of body parts (autotopagnosia)
Ask the patient to move on command and to name various parts of his body, to point to them and to parts of the examiner's body.

Unawareness or neglect of body parts (anosognosia)
The patient may ignore an injured or functionally defective part of his body, e.g. hemiplegic limbs or hemianopic field defect. He may verbally deny the functional defect or deny ownership of the affected body part.

Dressing difficulties

Does the patient show undue difficulty in dressing and undressing, get muddled when inserting limbs into clothing, or try to put garments on the wrong way round?

Sequential tasks

Test the patient's ability in tests of sequential hand movements, alternating tapping tests, alternating choice tasks, and alternating written sequences. These will have special relevance when a frontal lesion is suspected, along with tests of verbal fluency (p. 27).

OTHER GENERAL INDICATIONS OF ORGANIC CEREBRAL DISEASE

Note the ability of the patient to sustain attention during the above tests. Did he fatigue unduly easily? Was he able to shift attention readily from one task to another? Was there perseveration in the use of words, in simple motor acts, or in response to commands? Observe for difficulties with abstract thinking; test for this by definition of concepts, e.g. difference between dwarf and child, or interpretation of proverbs.

Note and describe any evidence of lability of mood, euphoria, or indications of catastrophic reaction. Were emotional responses exaggerated, flattened, or lacking? Did he appreciate his failings and show appropriate concern? Did he make use of evasions or excuses to cover up his defects?

8

Examination of the mute, apparently inaccessible patient and severely mentally handicapped patient

---

States of mutism, 'stupor', and apparent inaccessibility may be due to organic brain disease or functional psychiatric disorder. In all cases it is necessary to perform a detailed neurological examination and to assess the apparent level of conscious awareness (as outlined on p. 24) before considering other aspects of the problem. It is also necessary to bear in mind the possibility of underlying metabolic disturbances, like uraemia or hypoglycaemia, and physical complications of stupor like hypotension and retention of urine. Finally, it is important to remember that the patient's comprehension of remarks made in his presence may be good despite appearances to the contrary.

The definitions of these terms are not sufficiently precise to be used as the sole description of the phenomena they comprise. The following features should therefore be described separately.

1. To what extent can the patient dress, feed himself, and attend to matters of hygiene and elimination?

2. When aroused does he briefly become alert and verbally responsive?

3. Assess his response to graded stimulation (as outlined in the Glasgow Coma Scale on p. 25).

4. Are the eyes open or shut? If open, are they apparently watchful and do they follow moving objects? If shut, do they open in response to stimulation, is there resistance to passive opening?

5. Is the physical posture comfortable, constrained, awkward, or in any way bizarre? Does the patient resume a previous posture if moved or placed in an awkward or uncomfortable position? Are there any spontaneous movements or acts? If so, are movements meaningful; do acts display special meaning, possibly on a delusional basis or in response to possible hallucinatory experiences?

6. Is the facial expression constant or varying, alert or vacant, meaningful or unresponsive? Is there any physical or emotional reaction to what is said or done to the patient, or near him?

7. Examine the state of musculature: is it relaxed or rigid? Is rigidity increased by passive movements? Test for negativism, waxy flexibility, automatic obedience, echopraxia. Note evidence of resistiveness, irritability, or defensive movements during examination.

8. In the neurological examination pay special attention to evidence of diencephalic or upper brain stem disturbance. Observe equality and reactivity of pupils and note quality of respiration, look for evidence of long tract deficit in the limbs, test for conjugate reflex eye movements on passive head rotation.

9. After recovery examine for memory of events occurring during the abnormal phase, and for fantasies or other subjective experiences occurring at the time.

10. *Mutism* is a condition in which a person does not speak and does not make any attempt at spoken communication despite preservation of an adequate level of consciousness. It may sometimes be the only abnormality in otherwise normal behaviour. Is it elective, confined to some situations, or in relation to some persons but not to others? Is the patient himself disturbed by it as shown by gesticulations or evidence of distress? Does he attempt to communicate by signs? When offered paper and pen can he communicate in writing?

11. Distinguish mutism from severe motor dysphasia, dysarthria, aphonia, poverty of speech or psychomotor retardation. Is partial vocalization preserved, are emotional ejaculations possible, can simple 'yes'/'no' answers by given? Test separately for ability to articulate (whisper or make the lip movements of speech) and ability to phonate (to produce coarse vocalization or to hum). Can he cough? Does he speak very occasionally and briefly on restricted themes? Does he reply or signal responses to some questions, but only after long delay?

A careful history from informants may sometimes enable distinctions to be made more readily than from examination alone.

SEVERELY MENTALLY HANDICAPPED PATIENTS

For severely mentally handicapped people there may be a major impairment of communication. It is therefore necessary, as above, to eliminate pain or a physical illness as the precipitant of a behavioural crisis. The first sign of a developing physical or mental illness may be an exacerbation of pre-existing symptoms or behaviour. For example, at the onset of a mood disorder in an autistic person, there may initially be just an exaggeration of the autistic features. Pre-existing handicap (e.g. speech impediment) may mask the expression of typical mental symptoms. In this case, check for secondary symptoms, e.g. vegetative features (sleep, appetite, weight, etc.) when depression is suspected. The mental state may be difficult to define in detail, in which case the diagnosis must be based upon a balance of probabilities.

9

The assessment of the elderly patient

The assessment of the elderly patient is essentially the same as that of younger adults. There are, however, differences of emphasis that need consideration. Assessment is frequently complicated by clouding of consciousness, intellectual impairment, physical ill health, and special sensory impairment. As a consequence it may be necessary to obtain small amounts of information at several sessions, together with much careful observation of the patient both in the interviewer's office and elsewhere.

HISTORY

Since many elderly patients are either unable to give a history or can give only a patchy account, it is *essential* to obtain details from a reliable informant. Such an informant is frequently not readily available, but efforts should not be spared to seek one out. Thus, long distance telephone calls or visits to the patient's home and locality by the doctor or other members of the professional team may be required. Assessment of the patient in his own home is also invaluable in determining ability for activities of daily living (see below). Where it is impossible to obtain independent information the interviewer should look very carefully for *indirect evidence* of accuracy such as the sequencing and internal consistency of the patient's own history.

For any patient the history of the present illness is an account of changes over time, but for the older patient the precise sequence of changes may be crucial, for instance in differentiating pseudodementia from the dementia of coarse brain disease. In such a case careful attention to which came first — cognitive impairment or mood change — can elucidate the diagnosis. When enquiring about schooling, academic level should be as precisely determined as possible, since low attainment (Standard 6* or less) may indicate low premorbid intelligence as a contributory factor to poor cognitive performance. Conversely, cognitive impairment may be confirmed in a patient who performs at an 'average' level, but who obtained a scholarship from junior school.

EXAMINATION

Examination of the mental state should be essentially the same as for younger patients, but with particular attention to suspected organic cerebral disease. For this the procedure detailed in pages 23–31 is to be followed. Many elderly patients with dementia are unwilling to undergo formal testing and respond either with irritation/anger or with bland replies such as 'I don't pay attention to that sort of thing'. Such responses are usually an attempt to camouflage a disability and should be handled with tact and discretion. If the patient persists in refusing to answer, the interviewer should try to engage in neutral conversation, noting all the while any internal inconsistencies in the patient's responses which might indicate cognitive impairment. Where the patient permits formal testing, in addition to the procedure in Section 7, a simple questionnaire of memory and orientation such as the Gresham Ward Questionnaire or the shorter Felix Post Unit Questionnaire (see below) should be used and repeated at intervals as necessary. It is important to test activities of daily living (ADL). These include dressing, use of eating implements, handling money, and other everyday items. The patient's ability to find his way around the ward, in particular the bedroom and toilet, should be tested. Information about ADL and ward orientation should also be sought from nursing staff and recorded in the case notes.

Some elderly patients with profound depression deny depressed mood, but show other prominent symptoms — so called 'masked depression'. Such patients may present primarily with anxiety, hypochondriasis, hysterical symptoms or cognitive impairment (pseudodementia). Careful questioning as to symptoms of depression other than mood disturbance, e.g. suicidal

* Standard 6 was the penultimate grade at school prior to leaving at age 14 years (see p. 38).

ideas, diurnal variation, low self-esteem, guilt, sleep, anorexia, and weight loss, will help to elucidate the diagnosis.

Many elderly patients suffer from concurrent physical illness, and a thorough physical examination should always be carried out.

THE GRESHAM WARD QUESTIONNAIRE (FOR ELDERLY PATIENTS)

This should be administered 3–4 days after admission and the patient's answers recorded verbatim for every question. (It is also vital for subsequent interpretation to record the date of examination.)

General orientation

1. Where are you now?
2. What is this place called?
3. Where is it situated?
4. What day of the week is it today?
5. What month are we in?
6. What day of the month is it?
7. What is the year?
8. What time is it? (Allow 30 min either way.)

Maximum score 8. Score leniently for each question answered correctly.

Memory for past personal events

1. Where were you born?
2. What year were you born? (exact year to score).
3. How old were you when you left school?
4. What year did you get married? (exact year to score). (If unmarried, what year did you leave home?)
5. Where was your first employment? (Rough indication such as 'a family in Clapham, a factory in Leeds, etc.,' accepted.)
6. How many years since you were last employed? (If still employed: How may years have you been in this job?) 'Not since the war' or 'not since I got married,' etc., accepted.
7. When were you last in hospital? (1 point either for exact year or 'three years ago', or something like that.)

8. When did your mother die?
9. How many jobs have you had? (Rough estimate will do, but not with too marked deviation — such as 10 jobs if actual number is 15.)
10. When was your first child born? (exact year to score). (If unmarried, use the birthday of a brother or sister.)
11. What was the name of the school you went to?
12. How old were you when you got married? (If unmarried, how old were you when you left home.) Exact age required for scoring.

Maximum score 12. Allow 1–2 years either way unless stated otherwise. If patient never had any employment, do not score *both* question 5 and 6.

Memory for recent personal events

1. When were you admitted to this hospital? (date and day of the week).
2. How did you get here? (form of transport and route). Score 1 point if either correct; 2 points if both correct.
3. Did any body accompany you? Who? Score 1 point for correct answer.
4. Did you see another doctor before you came here? Score 1 point *only* if doctor's name given (GP's name does not score).
5. Where did you see him and when? (Exact name of place has to be given for scoring. Re. time, such statements as 'last month', etc., will do for scoring.) Score 1 point if either indicated; 2 points if both.
6. What is my name? (Make sure you introduce yourself to the patient once or twice during previous interviews.) Score 1 point only if exact.
7. When did I last see you? Score 1 point only if correct.
8. How many days ago did I take a blood test? (Or, did I take your blood pressure?) Score 1 point only if correct day is given.

Maximum score 11.

Memory for general events

1. Has anything important happened in the world recently? Score 1 point for important event, making allowances for patient's educational background.
2. Who is on the throne?
3. How many children has she got?
4. What are their names? Score 1 point for number and another point if all four names correct.
5. What is the name of the present Prime Minister?
6. Who was the Prime Minister before him/her?
7. What is the name of the President of the USA?
8. Who was the President before him?
9. When did the last war start/finish? Score 2 points if both years correct; 1 point for one year correct.
10. Describe the nature of one recent strike, accident, or national catastrophe. Where and when did it happen? Score 2 points if both reasonably correct.

Maximum score 12.

FELIX POST UNIT QUESTIONNAIRE (FOR ELDERLY PATIENTS)

Name: *Date:*   *Time:*
Age: *Date of birth:*
Education (ring appropriate category): diploma or degree/trade training or apprenticeship/left school at 14 i.e. standard 7/left school before 14 or at less than standard 7.
Case no: *Tested by:*
Tested at:

Introduce yourself and where you're from (e.g. Maudsley Hospital) at the beginning of the test.

Then say: 'I would like you to remember this name and address':

John Brown,
42 Church Street,
Deptford.

NB Substitute a more local place name as appropriate.
'Can you repeat it?'

If patient is unable to say it, repeat the name and address, and ask him to repeat it again.

Administer the following questions conversationally; the exact words used may be varied slightly to ensure the patient understands the question, but no help with the answers must be given.
Record the patient's responses verbatim in the space provided.
One mark is scored for each correct answer.

Comments:

	Verbatim response	Score
1. What year were you born?		1/0
2. What month are we in?		1/0
3. Who is on the throne?		1/0
4. What day of the week is it today?		1/0
5. What year is it now?		1/0
6. What is the name of the present Prime Minister?		1/0
7. Has anything important happened in the world recently? (Score for important event; prompt — what's been in the news recently, in the papers, on TV or radio?)		1/0
		1/0
8. When did the Second World War finish?		1/0
9. How old are you?		1/0
10. What time of day is it? Morning, afternoon, evening, night.		1/0
11. What time is it? (score if within an hour of correct time)		1/0
12. What season are we in?		1/0
13. What is this room called?		1/0

14. What's my name?   1/0
15. Where am I from?   1/0
16. What was the name and
    address I mentioned a
    .few minutes ago?   John   1/0
                                         Brown   1/0
                                         42   1/0
                                         Church Street   1/0
                                         Deptford   1/0

Total score (maximum 20)

-------------------------- 10 --------------------------

Eliciting and recording clinical information in child and adolescent psychiatry

INTRODUCTION

Sources of information

Children are usually referred as a result of adult concern about their behaviour. Assessment aims to get the best possible account of the child's behaviour and the feelings it engenders. Children never live alone at home and during the school years they are legally obliged to attend school. Their social and personal development is strongly influenced by the relationships and attitudes experienced in these settings. The pattern of these attitudes and the quality of relationships in the child's family, school, etc., require assessment. Much more reliance is placed on accounts derived from a variety of informants than is usual in adult psychiatry. A comparison of accounts of the child's behaviour and reactions to it at home, at school, and as observed during the assessment allow the problem to be categorized as situational or pervasive. There can be marked differences between reports from home and school. In general, pervasive problems are of greater psychiatric significance.

Mode of assessment

The child is continually developing. Symptoms and behaviours relate to developmental stages, as do emotional needs. It is very important to study the child's family as well as the child himself. Knowledge of the family may aid understanding of how the child has developed in the way he has. In some cases the most important factors in aetiology may lie within the family. In all cases an appreciation of the strengths and weaknesses of the family unit will be important in planning the child's treatment. It is also necessary to know what impact the child's difficulties have had on the family life, and how the parents and siblings have reacted. Every opportunity should be taken to observe the child's interaction with other members of the family and their interaction with each other, for example during introductions and while the programme of assessment is outlined even if formal family meetings are not undertaken.

Advantage should be taken of the opportunity to compare the child's behaviour across more and less structured parts of the assessment, for example in individual interview, with siblings in the waiting room, and during psychometric testing.

Several considerations influence the choice of mode of assessment. The nature of the problem may require a particular type of assessment, for example an individual interview with a suicidal child or psychotic mother. It may be appropriate to send other family members out of the room if marital sexual matters require discussion.

If the child waits outside the room while his parent is giving the history, there must be adequate play facilities and supervision, and he must be informed what is happening. Preschool children may not tolerate separation in a strange environment. The same considerations apply to siblings.

It is difficult to gather a traditional history with the whole family in the room. *Whole family interviewing* is a technique which generates a different type of information notably about live interactions, e.g. hierarchy, patterns of communication, affective tone, alliances.

A wide variety of techniques are currently used, but in most the interviewer takes an active role from the outset; engaging all family members, promoting interaction, and demonstrating that he values everyone's communications (even younger siblings).

Talk about the referred problem often starts a session. Discussion between pairs of family members may be used. There is variation in the extent to which it is recommended that historical data are brought in. Techniques include active employment of all family members in the construction of a family tree and exploration of the development of the parents' relationship.

If a particular therapy is envisaged then assessment in that mode is usually indicated. The way the various components of the assessment are ordered should be planned for each patient.

Interviewing parents

The history-taking consists of two aspects: (a) the obtaining of information about events, happenings, and behaviour; and (b) the recording of actively expressed feelings, emotions, or attitudes concerning these events or the individuals participating in them. Because much of the interview is concerned with eliciting precise factual material, it is particularly important to establish early on that the interviewer is interested in *feelings* as well as events. By expressing interest in the informant's expression of emotions and attitudes, the spontaneous production of emotional and attitudinal material can be increased. This can be done as well by the interviewer's general reaction and vocal, but nonverbal encouragement as by anything he says. Care should be taken to encourage positive and negative attitudes to an equal extent. Where the informant's feelings are in doubt questions such as 'does this kind of thing ever cause an atmosphere in the home?' or 'does that ever make you feel on edge?' are also useful, but should be used sparingly. In assessing the informant's feelings and emotions attention should be paid to the way things are said as well as to what is said. Differences in the tone of voice, shown in the speed, pitch, and intensity of speech, can be very important in the recognition of emotions. Particular attention should be paid to expressed criticism, hostility, and warmth, and to whom it is directed. Facial expressions and gestures should also be taken into account.

It is always desirable to see *both* the mother and the father. The child's relationship with his father is as important as that with his mother although the importance of each, to some extent, lies in different aspects of development. It is undesirable to have to rely only on a second-hand account of the father obtained from the mother. An interview with two parents together will often provide a good opportunity of observing parental interaction and relationships. If the parents are divorced or separated and the child spends time with each of them it may be more appropriate to see the other parent on a separate occasion.

Information from school and other sources outside the family

Parental consent should always be obtained to contact any agency other than the referrer and the family doctor. Permission to contact the school and other involved agencies can be requested when the first appointment is sent.

A teacher's account of the child's behaviour at school is indispensable. Ask for information about:

attendance;
academic strengths and weaknesses;
non-academic skills, e.g. art, music, woodwork, sports, etc.;
behaviour in the classroom and playground;
social relationships with teachers and peers;
any other observations of importance.

For preschool children a report along the same lines from a nursery or playgroup leader is of similar importance. It can be helpful to have this information available at the first assessment.

It is good practice to explain to the family that a letter will be sent to the family doctor after the assessment and request made to obtain old medical records, etc. The family doctor frequently possesses further essential information.

The child

The child is a most important source of information and must always be seen separately unless separation anxiety precludes this. If separation is not possible record this and evaluate it in the light of the child's developmental age.

The child's view of the problem should be sought. The sophistication of this view will vary with developmental age. Teenagers may be able to provide a complete history and often prefer to be seen *before* their parents, but their story must still be considered in conjunction with the accounts provided by the adults responsible for them (parents, teachers, probation officer, social worker, etc.).

The psychiatric examination suggested here may sometimes prove to be too full to be covered in the time available, especially with emergency referrals. In such cases the psychiatrist will have to decide what can be omitted *at the first interview* in the light of the individual problems. It should be realized that the diagnostic process continues in subsequent interviews and may intertwine with therapy. The *initial* assessment, should always include a systematic account of the child's behaviour and emotions, an assessment of the family situation, and an adequate diagnostic interview and physical assessment of the child.

SCHEME FOR HISTORY FROM PARENTS AND EXAMPLES OF
QUESTIONING

Referral

Note referral details and source of referral.

Present complaint

The interview with the parents should always begin with an enquiry about the problems or difficulties which are the chief cause of concern to the informant.

These are the focus of the attendance as far as the parent is concerned and a good deal of time should be spent on obtaining detailed information about them. The complaints spontaneously offered about the child are at least as important in their reflection of the parental attitudes as they are with respect to the main psychiatric problem exhibited by the child. In consequence, it is important to let the parents tell their story in their own words and, as far as possible, a verbatim account should be taken. When the parents have finished their account of the problem they should be asked if there are any other difficulties. This part of the interview gives a good opportunity to assess parental feelings and attitudes, and these should be carefully described. Only when no more problems are offered should the interviewer proceed with more systematic questioning.

The doctor should make clear how the referral was initiated (e.g. by the school, parent, etc.) and for what reason. If the referral originated from someone other than the mother or father the parents should be asked how they feel about it.

The parents should then be asked for a more detailed description of the symptoms that have been mentioned spontaneously.

Recent examples of the behaviour in question should always be obtained as well as the *frequency* of the behaviour, the *severity*, and the *context* of its occurrence. For example, does it happen at school or when the child is away from home? The circumstances which *antecede or precipitate* the behaviour and those which *ameliorate or aggravate* the difficulties should always be noted. In addition, the interviewer should find out what *strategies* have been used to deal with the problem, and how much success or failure they have had with each method. It is useful, too, at this point to find out what *effect*, if any, the symptom has had on the rest of the family. It is always important to determine the time of *onset* of the difficulties and the account should go back to the point in the child's development when his behaviour or emotions first appeared unusual, abnormal, or a cause for concern. Possible stresses current at that time should be enquired after.

If appropriate, the interviewer should also enquire what led to the seeking of help with regard to the child's problem and why help has been sought now rather than at any other time. (With school or court referrals the parents may not have sought help and may not recognize any problem in their child's behaviour.)

If delayed or deviant development is prominent whether global or specific turn to Appendix 2 — The assessment of children with developmental disorders including infantile autism and mental handicap.

SYSTEMATIC QUESTIONING

Recent behaviour and emotional state

General Health

Is he off school at all? Does he suffer from asthma, headaches, stomachaches, or bilious attacks? How good is his sight and hearing?

Speech

Does he speak as well as others of same age or have difficulty in pronounciation, a lisp, baby talk or stutter? *If marked difficulties, turn to Appendix 2.*

Eating, sleeping, elimination, etc.
Are there eating difficulties at home or at school? Does he show food refusal or faddiness? Pica? Does he have sleeping difficulties — poor settling at night, waking in the night, nightmares? What are the sleeping arrangements? Is there enuresis — diurnal or nocturnal? Wetting when away from home? Ever dry? Soiling? Smearing? Ever clean? Where is lavatory? *Regularity of function is also a temperamental attribute.*

Muscular system and concentration
Is he overactive or restless? Will he stay still if expected to or is he fidgety? Does he show clumsiness? Preference for a particular hand and foot? How good is his concentration and what is the longest time he can concentrate on something interesting? Is there any change or loss of interest?

Tics and mannerisms
Does he have any twitches? Where? Headbanging? Habits or rituals? Soft toy or blanket?

Attack disorders
Does he suffer from fainting fits or absences? *If the child does have attacks turn to section on the diagnostic assessment of epilepsy in childhood (Appendix 1).*

Emotions
Is he happy or miserable? Does he cry? Is he worried, depressed, suicidal, irritable, sulky? Does he show temper? Exhibit fears and panics? Tears on getting to school? School refusal? Is he fussy?

Peer relationships
(*Note: perhaps the best single indicator of adjustment.*)

Relationships with sibs
How do they get on? Is he particularly attached to any? How is this shown? Does he squabble and with whom? Do they come to blows? Does he show jealousy?

Relationships with adults

(Note: this is a convenient time to discover parental attitudes).
How does the child get on with mother/father? How is affection
shown? Is he an easy child to get on with? How does he compare
with other children? Whom does he take after and how? How
does he get on your nerves?

  *Children often have important relationships with adults outside the
immediate family. It is necessary to enquire systematically about these.*
How does he get on with other adults? With teachers? Is there
anyone he is particularly attached to? Does anyone help to look
after him?

Antisocial trends

Is he disobedient? Destructive? Fire setting? Does he tell lies?
Steal? Does this behaviour occur at home or outside? On his own
or with others? How is it dealt with? Has he truanted? Run away?
Does he smoke, drink, sniff glue or take drugs? Has he been in
trouble with the police? *If yes, obtain details.*

Sex

Is he interested in the opposite sex? Menarche? Body hair? Masturbation? Has he been instructed on sex? Does he ask questions?
Has he any sexual experience?

Present schooling

Which school does he attend? Does he like it? Progress? Reports?
Has the parent seen his teacher? (*See introductory section on school.*)

Strengths

What are the child's good qualities? What is the nicest thing about
him? What is he good at?

Family history and circumstances

Family structure and history

Describe appearance, manner, and mental state of parental informant(s).
  (a) Persons in home: *Obtain a list. It may be helpful to draw a family
tree.* Ask about — age, religion, occupation, education, health,
illness, personality, psychiatric disorder, seen by psychiatrist,
difficulty learning to read or speak, emotional difficulties,
enuresis. Have his parents been married before? Are the children

adopted or fostered? Mother's pregnancies — miscarriages, still-births? *Make sure biological parents are identified. Get the same details about a parent or sibs who live away from home.*
  (b) Grandparents and parental sibs? What contact is there and what is the child's relationship? Give details of the parents' own childhood.
  (c) Family history of psychiatric disorders, psychiatric treatment, depression, suicide, language delay, difficulty learning to read, enuresis, social oddness, alcoholism, epilepsy, court appearances.

Home circumstances
(*Note: A home visit provides the best quality information and can often throw light on puzzling aspects of the history*). Does he live in a house or flat? How many rooms are there? Are there others in the home? What are the sleeping arrangements? Facilities (bath, lavatory, etc.)?

Other care arrangements
Does anyone else look after him — grandparent, baby minder, neighbour after school, au pair, divorced parent at weekends, etc.?

Finances
What sources of finance are there? Are there any difficulties?

Neighbourhood
How long has he lived there? Give a description of area. Is it liked or disliked? Is there conflict with his neighbours? Is there any environmental threat, e.g. frequent assaults?

Family life and relationships
Parental relationships
How do they get on? What things do they enjoy doing together? How do they spend evenings and weekends? To what extent does the father participate in child care, discipline, and household tasks?

Parent–child interaction
What things done by child? Do they go out together? Play together? Help with homework? Help make things?

Child's participation in family activities
Does he help with dressing, feeding, etc.? Who helps? Is he taken to school? Does the child help with washing up, shopping, errands, etc.?

Family pattern of relationships
Is he the mother's child or father's child? Confide in father or in mother? What attachments to other adults are there?

Rules at home
Are there bedtime regulations? Does he climb on furniture? Leave the house without saying where he's going, etc.? Are there restrictions on friends, staying out late, reading or TV? Who monitors the child's behaviour? Who reprimands? What method of punishment is used? Does he have pocket money?

Personal history

A general account of the art of eliciting a developmental history is to be found in Appendix 2 on the assessment of children with developmental disorders, etc.

Pregnancy
Was it planned or not, and in what circumstances? e.g. adverse reaction of mother's own parents, abandoned by baby's father, half-way house. *Complications*: Toxaemia? Haemorrhage? Infection? Smoking? Alcohol? Drugs? X-rays?

Delivery
Home or hospital? Length of labour? Presentation? Mode of delivery? Maturity? Birthweight? Complications? Resuscitation required? Incubator or Special Care Baby Unit? Give details of the mother's health during and after pregnancy including depression.

Neonatal period
Were there difficulties breathing or sucking? Cyanotic attacks? Convulsions? Jaundice? Floppiness? Infection? Was he kept in hospital longer than usual?

Feeding in infancy
Was he breast or bottle fed? When was he weaned? Were there difficulties?

Sleep pattern in infancy

Social development in infancy
Was he placid or active? Irritable? What was his response to his mother? Did he cry a lot? What other attachments did he have?

Milestones
Sitting unsupported. Walking unaided. First word with meaning. First two-word phrases. Comparison with sibs.

Bladder and bowel control
When was he dry by day and by night (5 years). When did he have bowel control (4 years). Were there any difficulties? Was training used?

Immunizations

Allergies
Drugs? Food?

Illnesses
Was he ever in hospital — in-patient, out-patient, clinic, operations, accidents? Has he had any serious illnesses — measles, meningitis, encephalitis, fits or convulsions?

Separations
Has he ever been away from home without his parents or been separated while in hospital? Has he been apart from his parents for as long as 4 weeks? How was he looked after? What were the circumstances? How did he react?

Previous schools
Which schools has he attended? How did he get on? Why was he changed? Has his teacher contacted the parents?

Temperamental or personality attributes
It is not easy to disentangle the child's pre-morbid characteristics from the

present problems, but an attempt should always be made to do so. The child's temperament is frequently best shown in his response to new situations, new events and new people, but attention should also be paid to his mode of functioning in routine situations.

Meeting new people

What is his behaviour with adults? With children? Does he go up to strangers? Is he shy or clinging? How quickly does he adapt to someone new?

New situations

How does he react to new places? New gadgets? New foods? Does he explore or hang back? How quick is he to adapt?

Emotional expression

How vigorous is he in expression of feelings? Does he whimper or howl? Chuckle or roar with laughter? How happy/miserable was he before the present problems?

Affection and relationships

How does he show his feelings? Is he affectionate? Does he confide? What friendships has he formed?

Sensitivity

How does he respond to a person or animal being hurt? What is his reaction if he has done something wrong?

NOTES ON THE PSYCHIATRIC INTERVIEW WITH THE CHILD

The psychiatric interview with the child must serve several purposes. It provides details of history unavailable from other sources. It allows objective ratings to be made in a semi-structured setting. It is a diagnostic instrument and one of the major tasks at the initial interview is to determine whether the child has any significant psychiatric disorder. Observation of the child's behaviour at the interview may be very helpful in this respect. The interview with the psychiatrist is also an event of considerable emotional significance to the child. Even if the child only attends once, that contact may have a considerable impact and it is important that it is therapeutically beneficial. If the child has to be seen again, his subsequent relationship with the therapist will be influenced by the impression created at the first interview.

Confidentiality

Confidentiality still needs to be negotiated, particularly with adolescents. The procedure varies with the age and development of the child. The expectation is that the interview will be held in confidence. However, some secrets may have to be revealed to others.

At the end of an assessment interview it is good practice to clarify with the child whether there is anything he does not want mentioned. These confidences should be kept unless it is not possible in which case this should be made explicit, e.g. 'This is so serious I think your parents have to know about it — will you tell them or shall I?' If the child is being seen for a court report or social services assessment this must be made clear at the onset.

Some differences from interviewing adults

1. The child is *brought* — the reasons may not have been explained or they may be inaccurate. The child may believe he is going to be told off, taken away, kept, or hurt. He may be waiting for a blood test or operation.

2. The child is not the main informant.

3. The child may not answer any questions at all, no matter how experienced the psychiatrist. Sometimes children or even teenagers who will not speak can be persuaded to draw or play a game.

4. The experience of *uninterrupted* time with total attention from a sympathetic adult will be new to many children.

Setting

The psychiatrist will have introduced himself to the child when he first encountered him, probably after he has introduced himself to the parents at the start of the assessment.

With younger children the doctor should get down to their eye level by kneeling or squatting to ask them their name and how old they are. Care should be taken to acknowledge siblings who may be present.

There are great advantages in ensuring that diagnostic interviews with children of similar age are broadly comparable.

The interview room should be arranged so that only the objects which the psychiatrist considers will be needed are in view. The toys and games which are available need to be chosen with care so as to facilitate the types of observations which are of greatest diagnostic value. Observation of a child is much more difficult in a room cluttered with toys. For the child aged 6 or more it is usually preferrable to spend most of the interview talking with the child in the manner outlined below. With younger children and those with language or global delay there will need to be a greater reliance on non-verbal communication, and interaction will generally be easier if it occurs in a play situation.

With more mature children or adolescents the interview may often take more of the form of the adult psychiatric interview, but considerable modifications are still required since adults often come to the clinic because of their own concern over their problems. By contrast the child or adolescent is generally referred because of someone else's concern.

Observe the parent–child interaction in the waiting room when collecting the child for interview. How do the parents handle the separation? How does the child respond? Are the parents warm, critical, hostile, detached, or understanding in the way they talk to the child?

General advice

1. Be non-judgemental. This does not mean there are no rules; there are, but often they will not need to be explained.

2. Be prepared to specify limits — destruction and rage are *not* cathartic. 'That's not what we do here', 'I want you to stop doing that'.

3. Avoid long silences which can become persecutory, particularly for adolescents — some can be engaged in a game, some will respond to 'I wonder if. . . .'

4. Accept pictures if offered, and keep them safely for they will be asked about another time. Pictures should not be put in the place of honour on the wall, it will not be possible to do this for all the children who come and someone else may take them down.

5. Do not speak in an artificial voice — children are quite tone responsive.

6. Do not rush in with direct interpretations.

7. Do not let the child take toys out of the room. Sorry, these

toys belong to the hospital and there would be none for you to play with if you took one home every time.'

8. Warn about the end of the session 5 minutes before it finishes.

Common errors

1. To keep off relevant, but difficult topics in pursuit of a pleasant experience for the child.

2. To side with child instead of displaying constructive neutrality.

3. To lead a suggestible child into inappropriate answers.

4. To build castles in the air on the nods of mute children.

Engagement

It is customary to begin with a reintroduction and an explanation 'I am a doctor who helps children of your age with their problems and muddles' (not a teacher). The child is told that he will be returned to his parents after a talk. He is asked why he thinks he has come and corrected if necessary.

Children aged at least 6 years or so

The child will often be on the defensive, knowing that complaints have been made to the doctor about his behaviour. It is, therefore, usually unwise to make any mention of the complaints at the beginning of the interview. The doctor should make it clear by the way he behaves towards the child that he is *not* acting as a judge or as someone that is going to 'do things' to the child, to correct him or change him. He should show respect for the child as an individual and show interest in him, in what he says and what he does.

If the child is expected to sit down for part of the interview, restless or uninhibited behaviour will be more readily observed.

The first aim is to get the child relaxed and talking freely, to assess the relationship he is able to form in such a setting, the level and lability of his mood, his conversation, and any habitual mannerisms. In order to provide an adequate sample of behaviour, there should be at least 15 minutes of unstructured conversation with the child. The child should be encouraged to talk about recent events and activities, what sort of things he likes doing after school and at weekends, what he does with his friends and with his family, the games he plays and the things he is interested in, what he enjoys and what he does not enjoy at school, etc. He may also be asked about his hopes for the future, what he wants to do when he leaves school or when he is grown up.

Respond with interest, concern, or enthusiasm as may be appropriate (to set a relaxed and informal atmosphere, to try to elicit a range of emotions in the child, and to assess the emotional responsiveness of the child and the kind of relationship he forms with the examiner). The interview must be geared to the child's age, intelligence, and interests. If the emotional responsiveness of the child is to be adequately assessed, it is necessary for the psychiatrist himself to show a range of emotions (being more serious or concerned when asking about feelings of distress or worry, and more lively when responding to the child's account of what interests or amuses him).

The child should also be asked if he has any friends, what are their names, what he does with them, how he gets on with other children at home and at school.

Emotionally loaded topics should be pursued as they arise. The examiner's response should not block or lead away from expression of pathology or discomfort.

Next the child should be questioned systematically.

Open questions are usually preferable and multiple choice questions are sometimes useful. Specific examples of relevant feelings or events should be asked for.

Indirect statements — 'I knew a boy once about your age who . . .' may be productive. If the child accepts this convention there is no need to challenge it with statements such as 'this boy is you, isn't it?'

It is expedient to ease off topics that seem too threatening, *but the interviewer should return to them.* Does the child ever feel lonely, get into fights, get teased, or picked on? Is he picked on more than most other children? Why does he think he is picked on? Similarly, he should be asked how he gets on with his brothers and sisters. If he gets into fights, does he like fighting, are they 'real' fights or 'friendly' fights?

The child should be asked specifically about worries, ruminations, fears, unhappiness, bad dreams, and the sort of things that make him feel angry. For example, he might be asked, 'Most people tend to worry about some things. What kind of things do you worry about? Do you ever lie awake at night worrying about things? Do you ever get nasty thoughts on your mind that you cannot get rid of? Do you ever get fed up? Miserable? Cry? Feel really unhappy?' Suicidal thoughts should be pursued where appropriate. 'Are there things you are particularly afraid of? What about the dark? Spiders? Dogs? Do you ever dream? What about bad dreams? Or nightmares? What kind of things make you angry and annoyed?'

If anything positive should come up in answer to these questions, the psychiatrist should probe regarding the severity, frequency, and setting of the emotions (e.g. 'Do you ever feel so miserable that you want to go away and hide? Or that you want to run away? When was the last time that happened? How often do you feel like that? What sort of things make you fed up? Do you feel like that at home? at school etc.').

It should be realized that children are very suggestible and will sometimes produce answers that they think the doctor wants. However, the anxious or depressed child can usually be distinguished by his affective state when talking about worries, fears, feeling fed-up, etc. Although it is important to ask the child systematically about these issues, it is also necessary for much of the interview to consist of neutral or cheerful topics. Note whether the child spontaneously mentions worries or extends his answers on those topics beyond the questions.

The child should be asked to draw a picture of someone or a house and everyone who lives in it, and encouraged to tell what he has drawn. This provides the opportunity to assess his natural skills, his persistence and distractibility, and also his attitudes and feelings, in so far as they are expressed in the drawing and what he says about the drawing. Handedness and fine motor skills can be assessed at the same time.

To assess attention span, persistence, and distractibility, the child should be given some tasks within his ability, but near to its limits. The drawing constitutes one task, but in addition the child might be asked to give days of the week forwards and backwards, the months of the year, and also do some simple arithmetic (such as serial 7s from 100, serial 3s from 20, addition, subtraction, or multiplication tables). This is one situation in the interview where the child is stressed; emotionally loaded discussion is another. Tics and involuntary movements are often at their most apparent when the child is under stress.

Children aged below 6 years or so

While the same issues are important and the principles identical for all children, it is necessary to modify the form of the interview with the younger child. A play setting will usually be more appropriate for the child of 6 years or less, but depending on the maturity of the child it may also be desirable sometimes to use a play-interview with older children.

Games and toys should be chosen to (1) be suitable for the child's age, sex and social background; (2) provide an *interaction* with the interviewer, and (3) encourage communication and imaginative play. The psychiatrist should get used to using a small range of toys, for example, farm animals, colours, a doll's house with figures, plasticine. Board games like chess are not very productive. Imaginative games such as the *squiggle game* (making a drawing out of the child's squiggle and getting the child to do the same out of your squiggle), playing with family figures, etc., may offer the best opportunity for eliciting a range of behaviour and emotions. Where possible, the child should be seen without the parents. However, with very young children it may often be better to allow the mother to come in with the child first and then, after a short while, she can withdraw from the situation or leave the room.

It is important to allow the child to get used to the situation before the examiner makes an approach. Initially, it may be useful simply to let the child explore the room and the toys while the doctor makes a friendly remark or two, and responds to the child's approaches, but makes no approach himself. The speed with which the child may be engaged in interaction and the way in which the approach is best made will vary considerably and must be judged in relation to each individual child. An attempt should be made to provide some activity known to interest the child.

The play situation should be utilized to make the same kind of assessment with the older child, and where appropriate, the child should be questioned in a manner suitable for his level of maturity. Young children cannot be expected to give descriptions of how they feel or to answer complex questions with long words about abstract concepts. Nevertheless, many can explain what they do at home, whom they play with, etc.

Description of interview

In writing up the interview, the doctor should start with a life-like description of the child: his appearance (attractive or unattractive), manner, style of dress, etc.; how he responded to the separation from his parents, to entering the interview room and to the doctor's attempts to interact with him. The course of the interview should be outlined in relation to what was done, and what was said by the doctor and by the child.

The child's mental state should then be described more systematically under the general headings outlined below.

CHILD MENTAL STATE EXAMINATION (GENERAL APPEARANCE)

This should include points such as size for age, dress, grooming, prevailing facial expression, stance, etc.

Overall outline of interview

1. Child's adjustment to the situation: apprehension, emerging confidence, friendliness, disruption, age appropriateness
2. Brief content

Formal mental state

(Note changes related to topic under discussion)

Motor activity

1. General level,
   (a) restlessness: inability to remain in seat appropriately;
   (b) fidgetiness: squirming in seat, movements of part of the body whilst stationary.

2. Co-ordination.
3. Involuntary movements.
4. Tics: rapid, stereotyped, repetitive, non-rhythmic, predictable, purposeless contractions of functionally related muscle groups, can usually be imitated or suppressed voluntarily for a time.
5. Stereotypies: voluntary, repeated, isolated, identical, predictable, often rhythmic actions, whole areas of the body are involved.
6. Mannerisms: odd, stylized, embellishments of goal directed movement.
7. Posturing.
8. Rituals.
9. Hyperventilation.

Language
1. Hearing: sounds, speech.
2. Comprehension.
3. Speech/vocalization/babble,
   (a) spontaneity;
   (b) quantity — e.g. mute;
   (c) rate;
   (d) rhythm — e.g. stuttering;
   (e) intonation;
   (f) prosody: pattern of intonation and stress;
   (g) word-sound production: infantilisms, consonants omitted or substituted, dysarthria, speech defects consistent or variable (dyspraxic speech);
   (h) complexity: syntactic and semantic — length of sentences, vocabulary, use of personal pronouns;
   (i) qualities: echoing, stereotyped features, I/you reversals, other oddities (written example if appropriate).
4. Gesture: imitation/comprehension/use.

Social response to interviewer
1. Social use of language/gesture.
2. Social modulation and responsiveness to topics, e.g. praise, reward.
3. Humour.
4. Rapport: e.g. odd, aloof.

5. Eye contact: quality, quantity.
6. Reciprocity.
7. Empathy.
8. Co-operation and compliance, passivity.
9. Social style: e.g. reserved, expansive, disinhibited, cheeky, precocious, teasing, negativistic, shy, confident, truthful, surly, ingratiating, manipulative.

Affect
1. Emotional expressiveness and range (laughs? smiles?).
2. Happiness.
3. Anxiety, free-floating/situational/specific phobias.
4. Panic attacks.
5. Observable tension.
6. Signs of autonomic disturbance.
7. Tearfulness.
8. Sadness, wretchedness, despair, apathy.
9. Depressed or suicidal feelings.
10. Shame, embarrassment, perplexity.
11. Anger, aggressiveness.
12. Irritability.

Thought content
1. Worries, fears.
2. Preoccupations, obsessions, suspicions.
3. Hopelessness, guilt.
4. Low self-esteem, self-hatred.
5. Fantasies or wishes:
   (a) spontaneously mentioned;
   (b) evoked (3 wishes, etc.).
6. Quality of ideation/play.

Abnormal beliefs/experiences
Use adult section if appropriate.

Cognition
1. Attention span/distractibility.
2. Tasks:

(a) draw a person (note handedness);
(b) write name;
(c) give days of week;
(d) months of year;
(e) counting;
(f) addition;
(g) serial 3's from 20;
(h) serial 7's from 100.
3. Persistence.
4. Curiosity.
5. Orientation in time and space.
6. Memory.

Attainment

Reading, spelling, arithmetic are best assessed with standardized tests (e.g. Neale and Schonell for reading). If a formal assessment by a psychologist is not available then the child should be asked to read simple passages, to recall their gist, and to write a sentence about a previous event. The fluency, accuracy, and comprehension of reading are all important. This testing is even more necessary for children with disturbed behaviour or frustration in the classroom.

Interviewer's subjective response to child

Finally, an opinion should be expressed on whether (and how) the child's mental state departs from that expected in relation to age, IQ, sex, and social background.

CHILD NEUROLOGICAL SCREENING EXAMINATION FOR CHILDREN
OVER 5 YEARS

Children with known physical conditions or a history suggestive of a physical condition (e.g. epilepsy) should have a full neurological examination.

1. Inspect ordinary gait.
2. Ask child to mimic:
   (a) heel-toe walking;

(b) tiptoe walking (possible above 3 years, usually no asso-ciated movements above 8 years);

(c) hopping on each leg (hopping begins at 3–4 years);

(d) kicking a ball of paper.

3. Inspection, particularly of hands and face, for dysmorphic features, etc.

4. Touch fingers in turn with thumb. Test finger–thumb co-ordination bilaterally. (Most 6- and some 5-year-olds can do it. Mirror movements usually absent after 10 years).

5. Check for dysdiadochokinesis on rapidly alternating hand movements (pronation/supination 15 seconds each side).

6. Touch my finger. Repeat three times for each hand (pos-sible above 3 years, with eyes shut above 7 years). Note tremor, consistent deviation.

7. Stand up, arms out, fingers spread for 20 seconds. Age 4 upwards: look for choreiform (small, jerky, irregular) movements of fingers. Over age 6: eyes closed, mouth open, tongue out. Look for asymmetry and drift.

8. Close inspection of eyes including ocular movements. Visual fields to confrontation.

9. Check face and jaw movements and power — whistle, smile, blow out your cheeks. Note tongue movements, wiggle tongue, lick upper lip.

10. Child removes shoes and socks (check shoes for uneven wear):

(a) check muscle power and tone in arms and legs;

(b) check tendon and plantar reflexes;

(c) check feet for dysmorphic features;

(d) measure *head circumference* and plot on percentile chart;

(e) measure *height* and *weight*, and plot on percentile chart;

(f) Estimate pubertal status (Tanner stages described on reverse of percentile charts).

Observe how child puts socks and shoes back on.

11. Test hearing:

(a) name large toys at 1-metre distance in a quiet voice (laryngeal component) — ball, doll, car, spoon, fork, brick, ship — out of the child's field of vision.

12. Check visual acuity (well-lit Snellen Charts).

If abnormalities are detected the child should have a complete medical history and a full neurological examination.

Appendix 1

Special points in relation to epilepsy

Begin by asking for details of the *first attack* experienced by the child: age, circumstances, description, duration, how it was dealt with. Then get similar details about subsequent attacks.

Be careful to distinguish and obtain *separate descriptions of all different kinds of attack*. For each type of attack probe regarding the following points:

Pre-ictal

Precipitating events:
Are they through physical causes, illness, fever, etc.; psychological, any stress, or disturbance?

Timing:
Do they occur at any particular time of day or night, how long since last meal, etc.?

Altered behaviour or mental state before fit:
Is he irritable, restless, confused, apathetic, etc.; minutes or hours before the attack?

Patient's activity at onset
Do they occur while asleep, on wakening, awake; reading; watching TV; walking out into bright sun, etc.

Ictal

Aura:
What are the patient's subjective, warning experiences — ask the child whether he knows the seizure is coming and what he notices first (giddiness, noises, lights, smell, funny taste, inability to speak, feels frightened, etc.). If the child cannot describe this experience he may be able to draw it.

63

Course

What is the first event noticed (noises, strange behaviour, cry, fall to ground, motionless stare, etc.)?

Posture during attack:

Did the child fall, go limp, remain standing, slump back in chair, etc.?

Movements:

Which parts moved? Can he point them out? One side or both? Synchronous or not? (e.g. turning of head or eyes, tonic stiffening movements, clonic jerking movements, restless or semi-purposive behaviour, automatic or repetitive acts, fumbling, mouth movements).

Spread (march) of movements:

Where did the fit start? Did it spread anywhere?

Consciousness:

Was the child totally unresponsive? Aware, but unable to talk? Fully conscious and talking?

Colour changes:

Did he become pale, flushed, or blue?

Autonomic effects:

For example, was he hot and sweaty; cold and sweaty; salivating?

Incontinence:

Was there any incontinence of urine or faeces?

Injury:

Was the tongue bitten, etc.?

Post-ictal

After-effects:

Did the child return to normal immediately or go to sleep or become sleepy? Was he confused? Was there any weakness or paralysis of arms or legs? Clumsiness? Difficulty with speech? Change of behaviour or emotional state? Other symptoms, e.g. headache? Vomiting?

Duration of this type of fit
Was this first time? Most recent?

Frequency of this type of fit
Do they occur by day or night? How long has he been having *this* type of fit?

If not mentioned by parent ask specifically regarding the following
  1. *Generalized convulsive seizures*, e.g. does he ever have attacks in which he passes out completely? Are there movements of the arms or legs in any of these attacks — tonic/clonic or clonic/tonic/clonic?
  2. *Generalized absence seizures*, e.g. does he ever have a momentary blank spell in which he seem to be out of touch for a moment, but does not fall down, and for which he has no memory? Does he have any movements at all whilst this is happening?
  3. *Other generalized attacks*, e.g. does he ever have odd jerky movements (myoclonus)? Does he ever fall down suddenly without jerking or going stiff? (drop attacks)?
  4. *Simple partial seizures*, e.g. are there any attacks in which he has movements of the arms or legs, but does *not* pass out or lose touch?
  5. *Complex partial seizures*, e.g. does he ever have episodes in which he does not seem himself or does peculiar things?
  6. *Reflex attacks*, e.g. does he know how to stop an attack coming on? *Ask the child privately if he knows how to make himself have an attack.*

Treatment
Is this by family doctor or paediatrician? Which drugs are used and in what doses? (Calculate dose/kg/day — does it fall within the recommended range?) What side effects are there? Have *blood levels* been measured recently? What do parents do during the attack?

Attitudes:
Obtain parental attitude to the attacks. What did they think was happening during the first attack? What do they put them down to? What does the child put them down to?

Does the child have epilepsy?

1. *Differential diagnosis* includes syncope, breath holding attacks, sleep disorder, benign paroxysmal vertigo.

2. *Pseudo-seizures* are more common in children who also have genuine seizures.

3. Remember fictitious epilepsy is not uncommon. Obtain the name of someone other than the parent who has witnessed an attack and who can be contacted, e.g. school teacher.

Notes

1. Children who are suspected or known to have seizures need a complete physical examination.

2. If the child is asked to count to 100, hesitations may reveal brief absence seizures.

3. Starting anticonvulsants is a serious decision. If there is still doubt whether the child has seizures after a detailed history, consider asking the child to hyperventilate for 3 minutes. In susceptible children this procedure will induce generalized absence seizures in most, and complex partial seizures in a proportion. If a good history of generalized convulsive seizures has been obtained there is no point in doing this test. In view of the potential danger, this procedure should be carried out only under careful supervision including the availability of drugs and equipment for the management of status epilepticus.

Appendix 2

The assessment of children with developmental disorders including infantile autism and mental handicap

Having obtained an adequate account of the presenting complaints, it will be necessary next to obtain further information on those aspects of *development* and of *current behaviour* that are crucial either to differential diagnosis or to treatment. It is usually most convenient to begin with a chronological account of development. Rather than go immediately to questions of pregnancy and delivery, however, it may be preferable to start by asking the parents *when* they first became concerned that something might be not quite right with the child's development, and *what* it was that aroused their concern at the time. Particularly with a first child, the parents' concern may have been aroused long after the child first showed delays or distortions in development. So it is helpful to enquire whether, with hindsight, the parents think that all was well before they first became concerned and, if not, what it was that might have been abnormal. Having established the time and nature of those first indications of concern, it is generally easiest to go back to the time of pregnancy and work forward systematically up to the present time. All the usual questions on development are applicable, q.v. Most parents do not remember at all accurately when milestones occurred if they were within the normal range, but they are more likely to recall them if they were delayed. It is important to focus on that aspect first before going on to tie down the time more exactly. When seeking to date milestones reference should be made to familiar landmarks rather than to ages as such. Thus, for example, it might be appropriate to ask whether the child was walking on his first birthday, or when they moved house, or at the time of his first Christmas, or when the second child was born.

Particular attention needs to be paid to the developmental aspects of play, socialization, and language. With respect to the milestones of language it is crucial to be quite specific about what is being asked. Parents are very inclined to interpret all manner of sounds as speech, and especially as 'mama' and 'dada'. Consequently, it may be wise to ask very focused questions such as 'when did he first use simple words with meaning — that is words other than mama and dada?' 'what were his first words?'; and 'how did he show that he knew their meaning?'. In addition to the first use of single words it is important to ask about babble, the use of two- or three-word phrases, the use of pointing, gesture, or mime, the following of instructions, and immediate or delayed echoing. It is helpful to identify some occasions that the parents remember reasonably clearly and then to focus on what the child was like at that time. In doing so, an attempt should be made to determine what the child was like at about *2 years, 30 months, 3 years, and 4 years.*

Few parents think of socialization in terms of milestones or indeed in terms of specific behaviours. As a result, although the topic may be introduced by some general question such as 'how affectionate was he as a toddler?', it will always be necessary to proceed with a series of focused questions directed at eliciting information in key aspects of social relationships and social responsiveness at particular ages. Thus, for the 6–12-month age period it would be necessary to ask whether the child turned to look the parents directly in the face when they spoke to him, whether he put up his arms to be lifted, whether he nestled close when held, whether he protested when left, whether he laughed and chortled in response to parental overtures, whether he was comforted by being picked up and cuddled, and whether he was wary of strangers. Similarly with toddlers, questions should be asked about whether the child greeted a parent coming home, whether he sought to be cuddled when upset or hurt ('did he come to you or did you have to go to him?'); whether he differentiated between parents and others in whom he went to for comfort; whether he showed separation anxiety; and whether he could be playful, and enter into the spirit of to and fro in a teasing or make-believe game.

Precise questions are required to elicit an adequate account of the child's play at particular ages. Thus, to determine whether play was normal at age 2 years the clinician should ask about the child's use of toys and other objects. Did he recognize the appropriate use of miniature toys — as by pushing toy cars along the floor making car noises, or rather did he tend to spin the wheels, feel the texture of the paint, or listen to the sound of a wind-up car? Was there any pretend play — as with the use of toy tea-sets, dolls, etc.? Would the pretend play vary from day to day and would the pretend element be used to create any sort of sequence of story (with the toy cars racing each other, being parked in the garage, or being used to go to Granny's home)?

Having obtained a history of the development of play, social interaction, and language — with special reference to the first 5 years — it is necessary to obtain a comparably specific account of the child's *current behaviour* in these areas of functioning. Before proceeding to direct questioning on particular features it is helpful to get an overall picture of the child's activities by asking how he spends his time on return from school or at a weekend. Such a description usually provides a life-like portrayal of the bleakness or richness of the child's inner and outer world, and focuses attention on the activities and experiences to be asked about in greater detail. For adequate evaluation to be possible, it is essential that the specific questioning be based on a systematic scheme that ensures that each of the crucial areas is covered, as set out in Tables 1–4.

Table 1 Scheme for current speech and language

1. *Imitation* — of housework, etc.
2. *Inner language* — meaningful use of miniature objects, pretend play, drawing.
3. *Comprehension of gesture.*
4. *Comprehension of spoken language.*
   Hearing: *response to sounds*; response to being called by name; reaction to loud noises; reaction to quiet, meaningful sounds; (mother's footsteps, noise of spoon in dish, food being prepared, door opening, rattle etc.); ever thought deaf?
   Listening and attention
   Understanding: response to simple and complicated instructions with and without gesture (get details of examples).
5. *Vocalization and babble (non-speaking child)*
   Amount
   Complexity
   Quality
   Social usage — does he babble back to you?
6. *Language production*
   Mode: gesture, pointing; taking by hand; speech.
   Complexity: syntactical and semantic; length of sentences; vocabulary; use of personal pronouns, etc.
   Qualities: echoing, stereotyped features, I-you confusion, made-up words, other oddities.
   Amount
   Use of social communication: asking for things; to comment or chat to and fro; in reply to questions; mute in certain situations.
7. *Word-sound production*
   Any difficulties in pronunciation; consonants omitted or substituted; which ones; slurring; dysarthria; are speech defects consistent or variable; nasality.
8. *Phonation* and volume of speech.
9. *Prosody*: pattern of stress and tonal variation in speech.
10. *Rhythm*: abnormalities of rhythm — stuttering, lack of cadence and inflection; co-ordination with breathing.

Table 2 Scheme for current social interaction

1. *Differentiation between people* as shown by different responses to
   mother, father, stranger, etc.
2. *Selective attachment*
   Source of security or comfort, to whom does he go when hurt?
   Greeting, e.g. parent returning from work;
   Separation anxiety
3. *Social overtures*
   Frequency and circumstances appropriate or not?
   Quality: visual gaze, facial expression, and enthusiasm
4. *Social responses*
   Frequency and circumstances
   Quality: eye-to-eye gaze, facial expression, and emotions
   Reciprocity: to and fro dialogue
5. *Social play*:
   Playfulness
   Spontaneous imitation
   Co-operation and reciprocity, sharing
   Emotional expression
   Pleasure in the other person
   Humour
   Social excitement

Table 3 Scheme for current play. Play is a good guide to cognitive
level

1. *Social aspects* (dealt with already in Table 2)
2. *Cognitive level*
   Curiosity
   Understanding how things work
   Complexity: puzzles, drawing, rule-following, inventiveness
   Imagination: usually impaired in autism, ask about pretend
   elements, creativity, spontaneity.
3. *Content, type and quality*
   Initiation
   Variable or stereotyped
   Unusual preoccupations
   Unusual object attachments
   Rituals and routines
   Resistance to change
   Stereotyped movements
   Interest in unusual aspects of people or objects

Table 4 Scheme for systematic questioning on other symptoms

1. *Emotions*
   misery/depression
   worrying/anxiety
   fears/phobias
   anger/tantrums
2. *Aggression/destructiveness*
   to others
   to self
   to objects
3. *Social relationships*
   parents
   sibs
   peers
   other adults
4. *Conduct difficulties*
   lying
   stealing
   truanting
5. *Somatic aspects*
   headaches, stomachaches,
     etc.
   hypochondriasis

6. *Attack disorders (see Appendix 1)*
7. *Routine activities (in globally
   retarded children it is important
   to enquire about competence in
   basic activities)*
   mobility
   sleeping
   washing
   dressing
   eating
   micturition and defaecation
   sense of danger
8. *Habits, etc.*
   tics and mannerisms
   thumb sucking, nail biting,
     etc.
   obsessions and compulsions

The remainder of the history is collected in the usual way.

Index